When we are very old

Reflections on treatment, care and support of older people

Lorna Easterbrook

Published by
King's Fund Publishing
11–13 Cavendish Square
London W1M 0AN

© King's Fund 1999

First published 1999

All rights reserved. No part of this publication may be reproduced, stored in a retrieval system or transmitted, in any form or by any means, electronic or mechanical, photocopying, recording and/or otherwise without the prior written permission of the publishers. This book may not be lent, resold, hired out or otherwise disposed of by way of trade in any form, binding or cover other than that in which it is published, without the prior consent of the publishers.

ISBN 1 85717 298 1

A CIP catalogue record for this book is available from the British Library

Available from:

King's Fund Bookshop
11–13 Cavendish Square
London
W1M 0AN

Tel: 020 7307 2591
Fax: 020 7307 2801

Printed and bound in Great Britain

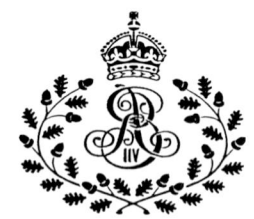

Contents

Acknowledgements

Executive Summary

1. Introduction 1

2. Quality of life – the aim of treatment, care and support for older people 3
2.1 Dignity, choice and autonomy 4

3. How far do current services and staff provide quality of life? 14
3.1 What helps …? 14
3.2 … and what hinders? 18

4. What is needed in terms of changes to services and staffing? 24
4.1 Health, housing and social care 24
4.2 Participating in community life 29

5. Messages for Government 31

6. Conclusion 32

References 34

Acknowledgements

The current and future treatment, care and support of older people was the subject of discussion at two King's Fund seminars, held on 26 February 1999 and 13 April 1999. Thanks are due to everyone who participated in the seminars for their willingness to share their experiences and views. Thanks are also due to King's Fund colleagues Penny Banks, Martin Fischer and Janice Robinson, who helped design and facilitate the seminars; and again to Janice Robinson for her comments on draft versions of this report.

Executive Summary

This report is drawn from two seminars attended by frontline practitioners and others working in health, housing and social care held at the King's Fund in February and April 1999.

Participants discussed their views of current treatment, care and support of older people, and what they would want for their own old age should such assistance be needed.

From these discussions, a number of key messages emerged:

- staff working in services are very critical of some aspects of current provision for older people
- there are major concerns about provision for the future
- staff have a great number of ideas for improving services
- there is no overall national vision shaping the system of support for older people.

For older people now, and for their own old age, participants want:

- treatment, care and support systems, services and staff that promote dignity, choice and autonomy, and enable older people to lead ordinary lives
- systems, services and staff that are firmly based on the premise of responding to older people's needs, as defined by older people themselves

- more adapted accommodation, and increased rehabilitative services
- multi-agency 'one-stop' information centres, covering a wide range of information and advice
- community facilities and public services better geared towards older people's needs
- key workers, to co-ordinate all aspects of treatment, care and support
- staff who can work across organisational and professional boundaries
- training for professionals to place greater emphasis on social and interpersonal skills
- increased support for staff.

Key priorities for change include:

- a decent income for all in retirement
- an equitable, transparent and reliable national system for funding long-term care
- greater valuing by society of older people.

Frontline practitioners are keen to see changes made and improvements implemented, and acknowledge their role in this process. However, not all changes can be made by practitioners, and there are clear roles for Government and others to play.

1. Introduction

Much of the current policy debate about old age is firmly centred on the role of the welfare state with regard to the provision of state pensions and the funding of 'long-term care'. In the case of the latter, this debate has been further stimulated by the recent report of the Royal Commission inquiry into long-term care funding for elderly people,[1] which recommended some major changes to the way support for vulnerable older people should be financed and organised. However, there is an additional debate that needs to be held in tandem with current discussions, in order to inform the values, aims and outcomes of decisions about the future of long-term care funding.

This report contributes to this additional debate, by focusing on the underlying purpose of treatment, care and support for older people, and by discussing the quality of provision for this section of the population. It is drawn from two seminars, held by the King's Fund in February and April 1999, for frontline practitioners and others working in health, housing and social care. Participants reflected on their current professional experiences of treatment, care and support for older people, and drew on their personal experiences as the relatives, friends and neighbours of older people in need of care. Both sets of experiences clearly informed their views on what they would want for their own old age, should treatment, care and support be needed.

This report does not offer a comprehensive view of current and future provision of health, housing and social care services. What it does offer is an insight into the views of frontline practitioners from different professions, sectors, geographical locations, age groups and ethnic backgrounds. Much of what they have to say is in line with findings from other research studies.[2,3,4,5,6] Their views both strengthen the debate about care for older people and add a powerful emphasis derived from the realities of directly providing treatment, care and support on a daily basis.

With the 1999 UN International Year of Older Persons drawing to its close, and a National Service Framework for Older People due to be implemented in April 2000, this report highlights what frontline practitioners see as the main aims of treatment, care and support for older people; whether they believe that current services for, and staff working with, older people are meeting these aims; and what changes in staff, services and wider society are needed, now and in the future.

2. Quality of life – the aim of treatment, care and support for older people

Discussions in the seminars centred on participants' professional and personal experiences of treatment, care and support of older people, and what they would want should they need this assistance in their own old age. The message from both seminars was unequivocal: the overriding aim of treatment, care and support should be the development and maintenance of older people's quality of life, now and in the future. Participants held clear views on what older people's lives should be like, but were critical of the extent of the failure of current provision:

'I'm not a bod in a bed – treat me like I'm a human being'

'I want a life, not a care plan'

'I want to enjoy life, not just survive'

'We must have services that enable ordinary life'

To participants, quality of life meant ensuring older people retain a sense of *dignity*, that they have – and are able to exercise – real *choices*, and have *autonomy* in their lives. They felt that services for, and staff working with, older people need to have organisational structures, training, management and political support in order to deliver treatment, care and support that meet these quality of life measures.

Perhaps more importantly, they believed that treatment, care and support must enable older people to lead the *ordinary, individual lives* they choose for themselves. In their view, a radical re-think is needed to ensure that society is better, and more positively, geared towards older people than at present; and that treatment, care and support for older people are placed firmly within this context.

2.1 Dignity, choice and autonomy

Dignity

One of the main ways identified as enabling older people to retain dignity was through sufficient income in retirement:

> *'Old age with resources is much easier than old age without.'*

Far from ensuring sufficient retirement income, however, the current level of state retirement pension was dismissed by some as derisory. Overall concerns about the loss of dignity because of poverty in old age abounded:

> *'How can it be dignified to have to choose between basic necessities like food or heat?'*

Many participants felt that ensuring an adequate income in retirement was vital. Even so, some had concerns that the normal costs of daily living restricted the amounts they were able to contribute to their own private or occupational schemes.

Concerns about the links between poverty and ill health in old age were particularly stressed. Not only are poorer older people more likely to experience ill health, they then often face what is seen by many as the indignity and gross injustice of having to pay towards the care and support needed *because* of that ill health. Payments due because of local authority charging regimes, including the national means-test for residential and nursing home care, were criticised by some as particularly undignified for the current older generation:

> *'I know it's been said before, but many of these older people not only fought for this country but they've paid for the welfare state which we – their children and grandchildren – have used. Doesn't that count for anything? If it doesn't then heaven help us when we're old, we haven't even got a war to point to.'*

It was felt that it is not only the *level* of income that affects older people's dignity, but the type, source and purpose of state benefits can also have an equally significant impact:

> *'Put me on benefits so I can access services – but don't put me on benefits that will stigmatise me.'*

Participants felt that some benefits are stigmatising. The manner in which these must be claimed is also undignified. They saw official forms as often extremely lengthy and difficult to complete, with frequently no assistance provided for completing them. In addition it was felt that older people are often reluctant to make legitimate claims to some benefits because of a belief that these are charitable handouts, to which some shame may be attached.

The low levels of state retirement pension and the concerns about stigmatising benefits were seen by some participants as symptomatic of the low value placed on older people by society as a whole. They saw this low value reflected by discussions about the funding of long-term care for older people, which placed too much emphasis on issues of affordability. They felt it is hard for older people in need of treatment, care and support to retain their dignity when facing attitudes, whether implicit or explicit, that they are somehow a burden on the economy and on their families.

Older people can also feel undervalued when their individual experiences, skills and preferences are not acknowledged; or if the trouble is not taken to find out what these might be:

'My biggest fear is that I'll lose my confidence and the ability to express myself.'

In contrast, participants believed that taking time to discover individuals' life histories, or helping older people to keep their memories intact, can positively enable older people to retain their dignity. Moreover, doing so is seen as an essential part of deciding to offer services which demonstrably reflect an individual's preferences, culture, religion, personality and life history, as well as any physical or mental health needs they may have. They would expect nothing less for their own old age:

'I'm not a bod in a bed, treat me like I'm a human being.'

Patronising attitudes and stereotypical expectations of what older people like to do and how they should behave were criticised as not conducive to people being treated in a dignified way, as individuals. This is not helped if professionals:

> '... are fearful of whatever's wrong with me.'

A lack of empathy, understanding and knowledge from professionals were identified as often going hand-in-hand. In addition, a lack of sensitivity as to whether individuals are literate, and in responding to different cultural needs, also affects older people's dignity.

Although there was a great emphasis on wishing to maintain independence, older people should be valued as individuals, now and in the future, no matter the extent of their abilities:

> 'I expect to be valued, even if I can't do a shirt button up.'

Remaining independent for as long as possible was seen as an integral part of maintaining both self-esteem and dignity. Yet, when independence is potentially threatened or compromised, treatment, care and support are not necessarily geared towards ensuring a dignified response and outcome.

Dignity is lost by, for instance, older people having to wait for assessments, services or equipment. An older person who experiences a delay of several months before a stairlift – identified by professionals as necessary – is fitted, might be forced to compromise on both their way of life and their dignity (for example by having to use a commode if an upstairs bathroom remains inaccessible). This loss of dignity could be compounded if equipment, when provided, was poorly designed, unattractive or showing signs of wear and tear. Some participants felt that this was again symptomatic of the low value placed on older people, especially those with disabilities or experiencing ill health, and that this was unacceptable:

'I want a stylish old age – give me a Conran-designed zimmer frame.'

Fear of accidents, fear of dying alone and fear of being forced to move into residential care were all cited as factors which adversely affect dignity. In addition, an individual's self-esteem can be significantly harmed if there is little or no support to help them come to terms with losses that they might experience when treatment, care and support are needed. Such losses include those of functional ability and of memory; bereavement – whether of partner, spouse or other relatives, or of friends; and losing pets, possessions and the person's own home if care in a residential setting is needed.

Some individual older people were identified as experiencing multiple losses, which, if support was not forthcoming, had an exaggerated impact. One example was of an older person who had been caring for their spouse or partner, as much else was also lost when the spouse or partner died. State benefits paid to the spouse, via the local benefits agency, ceased from the day of death. Any services from the NHS, social services department, private or voluntary sector would also come to an abrupt end. Equipment provided by the NHS or social services might be removed straight away, or could remain in the house for some time to come, both of which could be traumatic. In short, older people in this situation face multiple losses: of their spouse; income; regular contact with known professionals; and of being a carer as a focus of much of their normal daily living. The responses to this situation by these different agencies were not seen as necessarily based on maintaining the bereaved person's dignity.

That so many agencies may be involved was also highlighted as illustrative of the complexity of current systems of treatment, care and support for older people. This complexity was seen as not only making it difficult for older people to gain access to the necessary assistance, but also as having an adverse affect on their self-respect. The lack of consistency across the country in terms of access to, and availability of, services was also criticised. It was felt that older people should be able to rely on appropriate treatment, care and support being available when needed.

Choice and autonomy

Closely allied to maintaining and developing dignity were the issues of older people being able to exercise real choices and retain autonomy in their lives. Choice and autonomy were, however, believed to be compromised without the development of a greater number and range of alternative services to what was seen as the often too-stark option of going into hospital or living in residential care.

For participants, autonomy meant older people receiving recognition from professionals and organisations of their role as equal partners in deciding about, providing and funding their treatment, care and support – particularly when such decisions had clear resource implications for older people, whether financial or in the provision or receipt of informal, or unpaid, family care.

However, it was acknowledged that choice and autonomy also meant different things for different people. A key concern of one participant was that if their needs or circumstances changed, their spouse/partner should not suffer. The priority for another was to have her own space and not be left:

> '... banged up with my husband'

A third was positively looking forward to being able to be:

> '... a wraggled old hag'

and wanted services that would support this choice. Others would positively choose to receive or provide informal family care:

> *'My job's preparing me to be the carer for my mother.'*

Having choice and autonomy in any meaningful sense therefore has to involve finding out about, and responding to, individuals' views.

Autonomy and choice were also identified as older people setting their own individual standards rather than having another's standards imposed on them. One example was that some might regard keeping the house clean as essential, where professionals and organisations held a different set of priorities. Listening properly and responding to individual choices was vital:

> *'Ask me, don't tell me.'*

One way of enhancing choice is by improving the quality of services, particularly of care in residential settings. Having choice and autonomy also means older people continuing to have opportunities to take risks; to try new experiences; and to maintain existing, and develop new, relationships — including intimate physical relationships:

> *'I want to be able to eat chocolate, drink alcohol, smoke and masturbate.'*

For several participants, it also meant having autonomy over when to die, as well as how to live their lives. In addition, choice and autonomy meant developing systems which enable easy access to treatment, care and support, that are consistent nationally, and easy to understand. Such systems need to offer greater co-ordination of all those involved in the treatment, care and support of older people, through a key worker who acts as the single point of contact. These systems must also demonstrate a flexible approach to individual needs.

Individual, ordinary lives

For participants, retaining dignity, being able to exercise real choices and having autonomy in their individual lives also included older people being able to access fully the wide range of facilities and services available to the general population.

Facilities such as transport and shopping centres were seen as essential parts of ordinary life, whether or not individuals needed treatment, care and support. Public transport needs to be affordable and physically accessible, whilst shopping centres should be both easy to reach and easy to get around. Other local public facilities such as post offices and libraries also need to be fully accessible. Older people who receive treatment, care and support should be able to enjoy entertainment, events and places of interest.

Remaining independent for as long as possible was considered an integral part of leading an ordinary life. Support to remain independent means providing treatment, care and support that fits around the lives older people choose to live, such as when and where these are delivered:

> *'I want help to fit around me and the things I like doing, like going to concerts or visiting friends.'*

For some, an ordinary life would involve choosing to spend time alone, as well as time with other people. It should include taking part in activities which individuals find interesting and relevant, including culturally sensitive options. One example of a leisure activity which adults of all ages might enjoy is playing Bridge. If a Bridge club is affordable and accessible, and if arrangements for treatment, care and support are fitted around an individual older person's attendance, their desire to lead their chosen life could be met. In addition, such activities increase opportunities to mix with people of all ages, which many were keen to pursue:

> *'I want to enjoy life, not just survive.'*

Another integral part of ordinary life for some was being able to maintain their usual role within their family, and with a partner or spouse:

> *'I still want to be mum, and have my children visit me as their mum, not as someone they **have** to visit because they have to wipe my bottom.'*

Maintaining existing networks of family and friends was believed to be as important as developing new friendships and relationships. Contact could be kept up through visits or social events, as well as via the telephone and Internet, but these all needed to be genuinely available, accessible and affordable. Older people's involvement in community schemes, such as community gardens, was seen as both helping to develop a sense of community as well as assisting individuals to find or maintain a role in their community.

An ordinary life inevitably means very different things to different older people. As a description, it covers activities ranging from carrying out chores to having a social life. Living an ordinary life means any older person who needs treatment, care and support being able to access general facilities and services, enjoy new opportunities and maintain existing pleasures in life.

3. How far do current services and staff provide quality of life?

3.1 What helps ...?

A wide variety of services, professionals and organisations were identified as examples of treatment, care and support that can currently enhance older people's quality of life. Some are universally available across the country, while others are local initiatives.

Universal

- district nursing
- physiotherapy
- over-75s annual health check

Local

- rehabilitative services and approaches
- Hospital at Home schemes
- sheltered housing/adapted accommodation
- intermediate care beds which can be accessed from the community
- assessing needs at home to help prevent hospital admission
- community alarm schemes
- Home Improvement Agencies
- Crossroads – Caring for Carers schemes
- 'out-of-hours' arrangements for overnight nursing services
- 'one-stop shops' for information and advice

However, these services, professionals and organisations do not of themselves mean that the quality of life measures of dignity, choice and autonomy to lead individual lives are being met. Much is dependent on the quality of each service; the attitudes of individual professionals and organisations; and the aims and outcome of the treatment, care and support being provided.

Training, and the attitudes of professionals, can significantly affect the ways in which treatment, care and support for older people is delivered. Good care was identified as synonymous with work environments where managers motivate staff and encourage appropriate training and re-training. Opportunities for training to be shared across organisational and professional boundaries, as well as between sectors, were viewed as encouraging higher standards and greater understanding about working with older people. They also offer opportunities for a broad exchange of information, knowledge and ideas.

Where staff believed it was a privilege to work with older people with dementia, for example, their positive attitude led to the provision of a higher standard of care. That some staff are kind was seen as an immensely powerful tool which enables older people to retain their dignity – particularly because such kindness was strongly associated with valuing, and responding to, the older person as an individual. Recognition of different cultural and religious needs, as well as individual preferences, has been translated into offering a wider choice of food menus in all care settings – although some felt there was still much more to be done.

Particular services were identified as helping to maintain dignity by enabling older people to have choice and autonomy in their individual lives. A prime example was 'out-of-hours' services, such as nurse assistants who are available to attend to people during the night. Such services demonstrate a clear understanding that older people's needs do not necessarily fit conveniently into a traditional working day. Rehabilitative services and approaches could offer positive opportunities for individuals to maintain independence; a choice recognised as one that is highly valued by many older people. Examples include services that assist older people to avoid unnecessary hospital admissions and permanent moves into residential care, such as Hospital at Home schemes; and arrangements to assess individuals' needs at home. For those who do move to live permanently in residential care, a rehabilitative approach from care staff can enable individuals to maintain a level of independence, which, in turn, can also promote dignity.

Local initiatives such as a Crossroads – Caring for Carers scheme and a Staying Put Home Improvement Agency, were considered to play a vital role in helping older people to remain at home. They help by, for example, giving informal, family carers opportunities and time to pursue their own lives whilst at the same time giving the cared-for person a new 'family'; and by enabling older people to tackle housing repairs and adaptations. Short-term hospice care was also felt to be highly effective in supporting older people to remain living at home for as long as possible.

Dignity, choice and autonomy are promoted through services such as 'one-stop shops', which offer a range of information and advice. Such information centres were particularly highly valued when different agencies were involved, such as local benefits agency staff as well as health, housing and social care services, and where these centres also acted as a resource for the wider community. The availability of information and advice about transport, leisure and education opportunities in such centres is, for example, a practical way of recognising that any need for treatment, care and support is only one aspect of the ordinary lives older people want to lead.

Participants felt strongly that enabling older people to lead full, individual lives also meant having access to a much wider variety of services. Concessionary prices for, or free, public transport was seen as particularly valuable for those on low incomes, as were reduced cost 'pensioner meals' in local pubs or cafés. Transport services such as 'Readibus' or 'Dial-a-Ride' can offer door-to-door transport, and someone to assist if needed. Leisure and education opportunities can also provide a useful stimulus. A wide mix of such opportunities means that some individuals can positively choose activities specifically designed for an older age group, such as Saga holidays and the University of the Third Age; whilst others can choose to be involved in activities which bring together a wide variety of people of all ages, through a common interest. Access to a telephone and to the Internet – including the ability to pay for both – enables individuals to maintain active contact with family and friends, and provides further sources of information and advice.

Finally, the attitudes of older people themselves were felt to be significant. Older people's increased involvement in the planning and delivery of services means that their views are beginning to be heard more loudly. There was an awareness that 'grey power' movements are growing in the UK, and that more older people are prepared to speak out about their concerns. Participants believed that this involvement will continue to increase, and is a welcome sign of older adults challenging stereotyped and patronising attitudes:

'Each generation is different, but we're all increasingly used to being consumers with voices. I don't see why I won't be heard at 80 if I expect to be heard at 50.'

3.2 ... and what hinders?

Although there were many positive examples of a wide range of facilities, services and staff working to promote and improve older people's quality of life, a number of significant deficits and concerns were also identified. One of the most telling was the highly negative view taken by some frontline practitioners of current provision for older people – particularly given that this criticism was aimed at the services they are currently involved in delivering:

'I wouldn't want to be an older person in hospital'

'I hope I don't live long enough to need the services'

'I'd rather die in a ditch than go into a residential home'

Fuelling this view, and one of the largest overall concerns raised in the seminars, is the low status of services for, and staff working with, older people. Such low status is reflected in, for example, insufficient resources to meet older people's needs – a state of affairs which is also seen as indicative of the lower value placed on older people by society as a whole. Services for older people are felt to still have a reputation for being the non-glamorous end of treatment, care and support. Low value and low status affects the morale of those working with older people. It can manifest itself in patronising and disrespectful attitudes, such as calling older people by their first names without their permission, or indiscriminately calling all older people 'dear' or 'darling'. At worst, it also means that older people receive poor quality or substandard care resulting in, for example, malnutrition during hospital in-patient episodes.

Malnutrition was also seen as symptomatic of the impact of increased specialisation amongst professionals. For example, some hospital nurses do not regard helping patients to eat as part of 'their' job because this is not a 'nursing task'. Such specialisation could mean that professionals are a long way from any holistic notion of treatment, care and support for older people. However, these changes are not necessarily limited to individual professionals. Specialisation between organisations was also identified as having a negative effect in some circumstances, particularly when it is not clear which organisation, and which staff, are responsible for doing what. Concerns were raised that this lack of clarity is, for example, already causing difficulties over the development of rehabilitation services. Where responsibilities are unclear, care is not being co-ordinated. Equally importantly, a lack of clear-cut responsibility over decision-making amongst different organisations and staff was seen by some as leading to a lack of action in providing the equipment and services needed by older people. Moreover, when organisations and staff are unclear about the responsibilities each holds, they cannot give the sort of full and accurate information about services and opportunities that older people need if they are to be able to exercise choice and have autonomy in their lives.

Opportunities to improve older people's lives by linking with a range of community services are therefore being missed, and this is exacerbated by what was seen as a lack of skilled care management. Fragmentation amongst organisations and staff also means an increasing loss of knowledge about others' skills and services. For example, there were specific concerns about a lack of understanding of the range of services offered by advocacy schemes, and the circumstances under which these could assist older people.

If professionals and organisations find it difficult to obtain this knowledge and understanding, it is likely to be far worse for lay people, such as older users, to be able to understand and know about the range of support from which they might benefit. This was felt to be particularly true for older people trying to access treatment, care and support for the first time. Current systems are complex and can be difficult to understand, with individuals having to approach a range of agencies for different types of help: the local benefits agency office, social services departments, their GP, district nurse, and the private and voluntary sectors. Official forms were criticised for being lengthy, not always clearly worded and often requiring older people to duplicate the same information for different agencies. Older people often make the initial contact with these diverse agencies at a time of crisis or loss, yet for many it is as if:

> '... they're made to jump through hoops at the very time they are most ill, most upset, most depressed and least able to cope.'

Insufficient amounts, types and ranges of services were also seen as having a negative impact on maintaining and improving older people's quality of life. Too few rehabilitative services result in restricted access in some areas, whilst a lack of an overall rehabilitative approach means that some older people are:

> '... just being left to deteriorate further.'

Some seminar participants were particularly concerned about residents in homes where the care ethos did not encourage residents to continue to do as much as possible.

A lack of alternatives to hospital or residential care was also seen as severely restricting older people's choices and autonomy. Too often, older people are admitted to hospital:

> '... because there's nowhere else for them to go.'

Once in hospital, there is a good chance these older patients will develop ward-based infections, with their health deteriorating further as a result.

Some services were criticised for being patchy: either they did not exist in all areas so there was unequal access, or they varied in terms of quality or ease of access. Some primary health care provision was described as 'patchy', for example, especially for older residents in residential or nursing homes where there might be a lack of GP involvement. Whilst local initiatives can be positive, there were concerns that these are often not integrated into mainstream provision, and any lessons learned are therefore not assimilated.

Responses to emergencies might be limited to locum GPs and ambulance services, yet these are not always what is needed. Out-of-hours arrangements are often very limited, leaving older people to receive services when it suits employers to provide these, rather than at a time, day and place that fully supports the ordinary, individual lives to which they aspire. A lack of services and staff to check on older people who live alone is also a problem, especially if individuals' social networks are limited:

> '... sometimes all you need is a friendly phone call.'

Long waiting times for assessments, services and equipment further restricts opportunities to continue to lead the lifestyle of the individual's choice, and can have a detrimental effect on an older person's self-esteem and sense of dignity.

Continuity of care, and of care workers, was also a significant concern. Without this, older people can find themselves having:

'... to start again from scratch'

by repeatedly explaining their circumstances to, and forming relationships with, different staff from a range of agencies. Failure to share information between agencies, although raising issues of client confidentiality, was also seen as a source of frustration to those who found themselves having to provide the same detailed information on a variety of official forms to a range of agencies and staff.

Looking beyond health, housing and social care services, concerns were raised about facilities and services that older people valued but were simply not provided with. Shortcomings identified included insufficient help with gardening and decorating; and inflexible housing design which restricts adaptations and leads to older people feeling 'locked-in' to their homes, unable to get out and about, or to manage easily within the home.

However, even when older people are able to get out into the community, overall planning of community and public facilities and services are seen as frequently failing to respond to, and reflect, their needs. Public transport was identified as often overly expensive or physically inaccessible. Public toilets are often few and far between, are inaccessible or do not exist. Traffic light controlled pedestrian crossings seldom operate for long enough to enable those with mobility difficulties to safely cross busy roads. Uneven pavements add to fears that, even if the person can get out and about, they will trip over and hurt themselves. The closure of local facilities such as post offices, libraries and shops can mean older people facing long journeys to reach alternative services; journeys that are often simply not a practical option. Some felt that large-scale shopping centres are designed to involve having to walk a long way in order to reach all the shops – again, not always a practical or realistic option. Such an apparent lack of concern for older people's needs in the planning and design of these facilities and services further fuelled concerns that older people were undervalued, as citizens, consumers and as users of services.

Overall, participants felt strongly that there was a lack of a strategic vision for all older people, including those in need of treatment, care and support:

> *'I'm not saying other parts of the population aren't important, but there is too much emphasis being put on people being valued because they're working. And if you're retired, it's only about being a volunteer. What about those who don't work and can't be a volunteer because they're too ill and too old? Aren't they going to be valued?'*

Without a clear strategic vision, and a strong national lead, many participants felt that efforts being made locally by staff and services to improve older people's quality of life are being undermined.

4. What is needed in terms of changes to services and staffing?

'What drives us to improve things is what impacts on our personal life.'

In order for the quality of life of older people needing treatment, care and support to be enhanced, participants believed that there is an overall need for significantly greater valuing of older people. Higher status for those working with older people will help improve the provision of treatment, care and support. In turn, greater valuing and higher status needs to be translated into increased resources, more services and staff, and enhanced professional training.

Alongside these issues is an equally important need for easier and fairer access to treatment, care and support through a universal, simplified and flexible system.

4.1 Health, housing and social care

Services

Improving older people's quality of life means providing a far greater choice in the range and amount of adapted, as well as adaptable, accommodation. There needs to be a true continuum of provision, from remaining at home on the one hand, to residential settings on the other. This should not necessarily mean, however, that older people must face multiple moves from one type of housing provision to another as their needs for treatment, care and support move along this continuum. Rather, the built environment, and the funding and provision of services will need to be sufficiently flexible to accommodate a much wider range of needs than at present.

Increased numbers and types of rehabilitative services, and service approaches, are also needed in all care settings. The purpose of rehabilitation for each older person, and the aims and expected outcomes, need to be clear to all parties to ensure that rehabilitation is carried out with older people as active and equal participants, rather than something done to them as passive recipients.

The overall delivery of treatment, care and support needs to demonstrably enable older people to lead their chosen, ordinary lives. This includes, wherever possible, delivering care where the older person chooses to be, for example, whilst visiting a friend or attending a concert. The focus should be far more on fitting the treatment, care and support around older people's lifestyles, rather than an older person experiencing a lifestyle that could be restricted by illness, disability and by service responses.

Development of key workers, to co-ordinate all aspects of treatment, care and support and to act as the single point of contact for an older person, was strongly supported. There were different views as to whether key workers should hold some budgetary control, or whether the role should be closer to that of an advocate or an administrator. In addition, multi-skilled generic workers are needed, to reduce the numbers of different staff involved in the delivery of treatment, care and support. This was felt to be more likely to involve 'upgrading' some staff rather than de-skilling many. Organisations need to be able to offer older people some choice over which particular staff will be delivering their treatment, care and support. There will undoubtedly be some potentially contentious equal opportunities issues to consider if such a change is to be achieved, both from the older person's point of view and from the points of view of staff and their employers. However, participants felt that the potential for an issue to be contentious should not of itself prevent a service change. Rather, it may mean an increasing sensitivity to, and emphasis on, identifying and matching individual staff as those best suited to working with particular clients, users and patients within an equal opportunities context.

More imaginative respite care was also felt to be required, particularly in connection with maintaining established family relationships. One example was that respite care might best be provided through a care worker enabling an older person and his or her adult children to spend time together as a family, and not in the roles of cared-for and carer.

The development of more 'one-stop shops' was suggested, to provide a wide range of information and advice. Recognising the ordinary lives older people wish to live, and placing treatment, care and support firmly within that context, means that such services need to be able to offer information and advice which goes beyond health, housing and social care services, and state benefits, to include broader financial advice, information on leisure and education opportunities, accessible buildings, and shops and transport.

Staff and training

The need for person-centred care delivered by person-centred workers requires that such an approach be fully understood and incorporated into the ethos of training for the full range of staff. Greater and more effective team working must be matched by training, both pre-qualification and subsequent job-related education, which identifies and develops necessary skills such as negotiation and mediation. Technical know-how is, of course, essential, but there was also a heartfelt plea for professionals:

> '... to have some personal charm.'

Participants felt it was important for staff to have effective social and interpersonal skills, and that this should be reflected in both the recruitment and training of staff. It was thought that this emphasis on personal skills, together with a higher status for older people generally, and for those working with them, would help staff to resist the stereotyping of all older people. Equally, staff were thought to need support through training, as well as through management style and workplace ethos, to enable them to deal with older people who were angry or distressed:

> 'I want to be able to be angry if that's how I feel – but staff need to know how to let me be angry without it taking its toll on them.'

Far greater acknowledgement is also needed of the potential impact on staff when their working relationships with individual older people come to an end, and practical steps should be put into place to support staff through this change. Whilst many staff took positive steps to enable older people to continue to take risks, others were reluctant or lacked the necessary skills to do so. Training and support for staff should, in this respect, take place alongside older people's views on what risk-taking means for them; and needs to be firmly placed in the context of a full and frank discussion amongst all parties about the extent and range of professional liability.

Identifying, recognising and valuing the skills and experiences of older people are all vital components of responding to individual needs. Many professionals would be concerned at any suggestions that they were not already doing so, or may argue that it is the systems of treatment, care and support that limit their abilities to provide services which demonstrably put these principles into practice. A much greater understanding of how these principles can be translated and integrated into practical support is needed, and older people should be involved fully in working towards this end. In the meantime, however, participants felt that individual staff could begin to take some practical steps:

> '... we all need to practice what we preach on a daily basis.'

If those currently working with older people wanted to be regarded as individuals in their own old age, there is a need for them to behave toward the current older generation in this way. Countering stereotyped and patronising views wherever possible, and acting as role models for younger or less experienced staff are ways in which individual professionals can promote change:

> 'Some of the people who will look after us in our old age are our younger, junior colleagues. If we want them to treat us with respect when we are very old, we've got to instil into them now that older people should be valued.'

Systems, services and staff

Systems were seen to set the context for services and staff, and change at all three levels was felt to be necessary in order to improve older people's quality of life in the ways identified by participants. For example, unless assumptions – whether explicit or implicit – that relatives, neighbours or friends will provide care change at the system level, it will remain extremely difficult in practice for service and staff assumptions to also move away from this view. Staff and services may be keen to develop the concept of older people as equal partners with whom they work jointly to achieve the best possible individual outcome, but may find their efforts are stifled without this being the basic premise behind systems of treatment, care and support.

Communication between systems, services and staff and with older people therefore need to be enhanced. Some participants felt that although the increasing emphasis on listening to older people at a service level was positive, this message needs to be adopted strategically and nationally. Listening is not enough: staff, services and systems all need to be able to demonstrate that these messages have been heard and are being responded to in practical ways.

4.2 Participating in community life

Many participants identified older people as a significant group of consumers and citizens, towards whom facilities and services should be geared, thus enhancing opportunities for participation in community life. They thought it vital that services such as transport be accessible and affordable to older people; and that the wider built environment be designed and maintained with older people's safety in mind. Measures which assist older people to feel safe in their own homes were also viewed as important, including, for example, tackling the fear of crime; of being taken ill or having an accident and not being able to call for help; and of dying alone.

A more inclusive approach to the organisation of entertainment and events was proposed, providing opportunities to mix with all ages. At the same time, those involved in planning and running such events should, if needed, identify and adapt to the interests of an older generation, building such interests into their planning and design strategies. Overall, participants believe that more community facilities are needed which are able to respond to an increasingly ageing population.

5. Messages for Government

A great number of the messages from the seminars are pertinent to central government policies, including those related to resource allocation and service quality standards. However, participants ranked two themes higher than any others as requiring urgent Government action. The first focussed on the need for a decent retirement income for all; and the second on a more equitable, transparent and reliable national system for the funding, provision and delivery of long-term care.

A third, overarching, message was the need for older people to be listened to, responded to, and valued. Within wider society, as well as within the funding, provision and delivery of long-term care, the Government was urged to lead the way, so that listening, responding and valuing older people becomes second nature to everyone. In doing so, the Government will need to specifically make clear how it will listen to, respond to and value those older people who are in need of treatment, care and support. Without this, the Government will be unable to develop and promote the overall strategic vision that is, in the view of seminar participants, both missing and needed as a matter of urgency.

6. Conclusion

Much of the content of the seminar discussions covers familiar territory. But it should be a serious concern that it is current practitioners who are critical of the services with which they are involved as professionals, or from their personal experiences of treatment, care and support for older relatives or friends. Many are dismayed and angry about current systems and services for older people, and have significant worries about their own old age, and for older relatives, should care be needed. However, they also have clear views about what constitutes good practice, and could readily identify services that positively promote older people's quality of life.

Many local initiatives have been highly successful, but there appear to be significant difficulties in adapting the lessons from innovative projects to mainstream provision. If there are barriers preventing this from happening, detailed investigation and analysis is needed in order to begin to break these down. Further analysis is also needed of the gap between an individual practitioner's passion for ensuring older people's needs are met, and what seems to happen in some cases in practice. This includes identifying what makes good practitioners, and what makes others apparently dismissive of older people's views, preferences and concerns. The ways in which practitioners and services relate to older people in need of treatment, care and support should not be distant or distinct from policy and the strategic view, but there is an overwhelming need to translate policy into practice from frontline workers upwards, and from strategists down. Achieving this is likely to be one of the next main challenges in securing improvements in the treatment, care and support of current and future older people.

Practitioners are keen to see change happen and improvements take place. However, they know it is not entirely in their hands, and that Government and others have a strong part to play in getting treatment, care and support for older people right, for this generation and the next.

Day-to-day practice could be much improved by better training, better management and increased resources; but what stands out from these seminars is the lack of an overall vision for support of older people. This results in an absence of a strategic direction for enhancing provision. What is found instead is a hotchpotch of innovation and good practice coupled with instances of poor standards, neglect and incompetence.

There is an overwhelming need to enhance society's views and opinions of older people and their role in society, to move away from arguably ingrained beliefs that they are a burden, towards a recognition of the value of their skills and experiences. Increases in the numbers of older people, now and in the future, mean they are becoming more visible within society. As a significant section of the adult population, and as major users of health, housing and social care services, older people have arguably been 'seen but not heard' for too long.

Changing attitudes, services, systems and responses now should mean improvements for those older people who currently need treatment, care and support, as well as ensuring a better outcome for those of us who may need such assistance in the future, when we are very old.

References

1. Cm.4192-I. *With Respect to Old Age.* London: Stationery Office, 1999.

2. Henwood M and Waddington E. *Expecting the Worst? Views on the future of long-term care.* London: Help the Aged, 1998.

3. Harding T. *A Life Worth Living: the independence and inclusion of older people.* London: Help the Aged, 1997.

4. Farrell C, Robinson J and Fletcher P. *A New Era for Community Care? What people want from health, housing and social care.* London: King's Fund, 1999.

5. Henwood M, Lewis H and Waddington E. *Listening to Users of Domiciliary Care Services: developing and monitoring quality standards.* Leeds: Nuffield Institute for Health, 1998.

6. Henwood M, Editor. *Our Turn Next: a fresh look at home support services for older people.* Leeds: Nuffield Institute for Health, 1997.